Dr.

MW00618575

24
Realistic Ways
to Improve
Your Health

Tim Arnott, M.D.

LIFESTYLE CENTER
OF AMERICA

Pacific Press® Publishing Association
Nampa, Idaho
Oshawa, Ontario, Canada
www.pacificpress.com

Copyright © 2004 by
Lifestyle Center of America

Published by Pacific Press® Publishing Association
Printed in the United States of America
All Rights Reserved

Additional copies of this book may be purchased at
www.adventistbookcenter.com

ISBN 13: 978-0-8163-2029-5
ISBN 10: 0-8163-2029-2

10 11 12 13 14 · 9 8 7 6 5

Contents

CHAPTER 1

Exercise the Right Way

When it comes to exercise, "no pain, no gain" is a myth. With interval training, also called intermittent training, you can actually increase the "gain" and decrease the "pain" of exercise significantly.

Interval training is a type of exercise that incorporates intense exercise with short bouts of rest. Here's how to do it. Find the exercising heart rate—beats per minute—that's right for you. Then exercise at a level that raises your heart rate five beats per minute *above* that comfort level. At that point, slow down to let your heart rate *drop* ten beats per minute. When that happens, exercise more intensively so that your heart rate goes back up ten beats per minute. Repeat this cycle up and down. As you do so, you will be able to keep your muscles burning oxygen and reduce the risk of overworking them. Overworked muscles build up lactic acid, which tires you more quickly and makes exercise become drudgery. Also, lactic acid buildup may decrease the benefits of exercise, even reducing the amount of fat your body burns during exercise.

Dr. Harold Mayer, while an exercise physiologist at Lifestyle Center of America, discovered that when individuals adopt an interval training exercise program, they lose more weight than do those who exercise using continuous training. In fact, in his study, the interval training group lost *twice* as much weight in just ten weeks as did those doing continuous training. Furthermore, those using interval training lost more body fat than those who used continuous training exercise. Specifically, those using interval training decreased body fat by 1.5 percent—compared to a negligible reduction in body fat among those opting for continuous training. Interval training may actually help you lose *more* weight and leave you with energy to spare compared to continuous forms of exercise.

If you don't want to bother with monitoring heart rate and counting beats, an easy way to do interval training is to choose gardening for exercise. While gardening, you naturally exert, rest, exert, then rest. Another simple option is to walk up and down hills. Such exercise choices provide an important way to help prevent muscles from working too hard.

Of course, if you're using a treadmill or other exercise equipment, use a heart rate monitor to follow the interval training exercise program described above. The important thing is to find the exercise program that works best for you—one you are most likely to continue the rest of your life. Even more important than how you exercise is the fact that you do exercise. We were made for movement.

Consider these important benefits of exercise. Dr. Frank Hu and colleagues at the Harvard School of Public Health discovered that women with diabetes who exercise have a lower risk of heart attack.[1] In fact, in his study, the risk was 44 percent lower for those who were most active compared with those who exercised least! The same study showed a 26 percent lower risk of type 2 diabetes[2] and a 40 percent lower risk of stroke for those who were most active compared to those who were least active.[3] Women walking about three-and-a-half miles per hour had half the risk of stroke compared to those walking less than two miles per hour.[4]

According to the World Health Organization, sixty minutes a day of exercise is about the duration required for weight control.[5] If you are unable to exercise for a total of an hour per day, gradually work toward this goal. Brisk exercise—about three-and-a-half miles per hour, if you're walking—is most protective of your health. However, listen to your joints; listen to your chest! Be careful not to overwork your heart or joints. If pain develops in either, see your physician immediately! Work closely with your doctor to be certain you are not exercising at an intensity or a duration that is dangerous. If you are over fifty years old, excessively overweight, or have diabetes, heart disease, high cholesterol, or high blood pressure, see a physician before starting an exercise program! Remember, if you are so out of breath during exercise that you can no longer talk to someone next to you, you are exercising too hard.

[1] F. B. Hu, "Physical Activity and Risk for Cardiovascular Events in Diabetic Women," *Ann Intern Med.*, 2001, 134:96-105.

[2] F. B. Hu, "Walking Compared With Vigorous Physical Activity and Risk of Type 2 Diabetes in Women: A Prospective Study," *Journal of the American Medical Association*, 1999, 282:1433-1439.

[3] F. B. Hu, "Physical Activity and Risk of Stroke in Women," *Journal of the American Medical Association*, 2000, 283:2961-2967.

[4] Ibid.

[5] World Health Organization, "Annual Global Move for Health Initiative: A Concept Paper," Noncommunicable Diseases and Mental Health Promotion, 2003, p. 6.

CHAPTER 2

Proper Rest Is Important

If you suffer from diabetes or want to minimize your risk of ever developing the disease, if you suffer from insulin resistance, or if you simply want to improve memory, rest is your friend.

Proper rest is important if you want to avoid diabetes. Dr. Spiegel of the University of Chicago found that healthy young men had 40 percent lower blood sugar uptake by their tissues when they got only four hours of sleep for six consecutive nights than when they had six nights of adequate rest. Further, insulin released from the pancreas was 30 percent lower after sleep deprivation than after nearly a week of adequate rest. And the ability of blood sugar to enter body cells without help from insulin dropped 30 percent, to a level seen in type 2 diabetes. In short, sleep deprivation left healthy young men with an ability to handle blood sugar comparable to that of an elderly person with a mild form of diabetes.[1] One explanation is that loss of sleep appears to raise stress hormone levels, which in turn may increase the body's resistance to insulin, leading to more difficulty bringing blood sugar into tissues.[2]

Proper rest is also needed for optimal memory. Dr. Fischer and colleagues at the University of Lubeck in Germany found that healthy young people were able to do a finger-tapping exercise 33 percent faster and with 30 percent fewer errors when they got a full night's sleep than when they went without rest for a comparable period of time.[3] The conclusion? Sleep is required to achieve optimal performance when learning a motor skill such as playing a musical instrument.

Similar findings were reported by Dr. Walker and colleagues at Harvard Medical School. They found that a group of people, taught to type a sequence of keys on a keyboard, were able to do so 20 percent faster and without loss of accuracy after a good night's sleep than when they tried to repeat the sequence after a similar passage of time without sleep.[4]

At Lifestyle Center of America, I recommend the following to patients wanting to obtain optimal rest:

- ◆ Rest seven to eight hours each night.
- ◆ Get two-and-a-half to three hours of sleep before midnight. Every hour of rest before midnight is equivalent to two hours after midnight.
- ◆ Consider leaving off supper or having only northern fruit, a plate of above-the-ground steamed vegetables, or a light soup in the evening. An empty stomach when you lie down to sleep will maximize sleep quality.

In addition, get thirty minutes of bright sunlight (or light box exposure) every morning, walk briskly for a *total* of sixty minutes a day, six days a week, and abstain from stimulating beverages, including alcohol and caffeine.

As a final note, if you have been told that you snore *and* find yourself having a hard time staying awake, or even dozing off, during the day, you may be suffering from obstructive sleep apnea. Talk with your physician about a sleep study. Weight loss can help reduce episodes of sleep apnea.

Rest is powerful medicine. Make time for it!

[1] K. Spiegel, "Impact of Sleep Debt on Metabolic and Endocrine Function," *The Lancet,* October 23, 1999, 354 (9188):1435-1439.

[2] G. Lac, "Elevated Salivary Cortisol Levels as a Result of Sleep Deprivation in a Shift Worker," *Occupational Medicine,* March 2003, 53 (2):143-145. R. Rosamond, "Stress Induced Disturbances of the HPA Axis: A Pathway to Type 2 Diabetes?" *Medical Science Monitor,* February 2003, 9 (2):RA 35-39.

[3] S. Fischer, "Sleep Forms Memory for Finger Skills," Proc National Academy of Science, September 3, 2002, 99 (18):11987-11991.

[4] M. P. Walker, "Practice With Sleep Makes Perfect: Sleep-Dependent Motor Skill Learning," *Neuron,* July 3, 2002:205-211.

CHAPTER 3

Spend Time in the Light

I once talked with a lady who told me, "I have been suffering with depression for two years." As we talked, I discovered she wasn't always depressed. She noted that after being exposed to as little as an hour or so of sunlight on the weekends, her depression left.

Why is sunlight so important? Scientists have discovered that sunlight, registered through the eyes, increases serotonin in the brain. We need serotonin to feel in a good mood and to help resolve depression.

Dr. Lambert at the Baker Heart Research Institute, Melbourne, Australia, found that the amount of serotonin in the blood carried by the jugular vein to be eight times greater on a bright day than a dull day.[1] Its important to note that the light intensity indoors with artificial lighting is often less than that experienced outside on a dull day. Most of us spend nearly all our time inside, thus, perpetually experiencing much lower light intensity than we would if we were outside even on a dull day. As a result, our brain serotonin levels may drop significantly. Additionally, the brain appears to make significantly more serotonin in the summer compared to winter. In the summertime, the blood coming from the brain has seven times more serotonin than it has in the winter under similar conditions. Sunlight in summer is of greater intensity than in winter, and more intense light entering the eyes stimulates greater manufacture of serotonin.

What does all this mean? If you have been suffering with depression and/or lack of energy, these symptoms may improve as you increase your exposure to sunlight. If possible, get at least thirty minutes of bright sunlight first thing in the morning. Morning sunlight is most beneficial. However, even walking outside during a fifteen-minute break morning and afternoon will also help raise serotonin. Make a habit of spending more time outside every day. If you have limited time, try to go outside when the sunlight is most intense.

The increase in serotonin in your brain is automatic and immediate upon exposure to sunlight. However, the serotonin your body makes today will not last until tomorrow, so you need outdoor sunlight exposure daily! On cloudy days and during winter, spend more time outside because light intensity is reduced.

Be careful never to burn your skin or even to turn it pink. It is sunlight entering your eyes that raises serotonin; your skin can remain completely covered. Of course, never look directly at the sun and always follow your doctor's recommendation about sunlight exposure.

Even if you don't suffer from depression, sunlight is essential to good health—both mental and physical. Make sure you get enough sunshine!

[1] G. W. Lambert, "Effect of Sunlight and Season on Serotonin Turnover In the Brain," *The Lancet,* December 7, 2002, 36 (9348):1840-1842.

CHAPTER 4

Water Your Heart

Linda was suffering with dry eyes. She had suffered a long time. She used eye drops daily. Then, she came to Lifestyle Center of America, and within a few days, her problem with dry eyes completely resolved itself. Why? During our nineteen-day program she began drinking more water. Generous water intake solved her dry eye problem.

Not only is water effective for a simple problem like dry eyes, but it is also powerful medicine for the most important disease in this country—coronary artery disease. Jackie Chan at the Loma Linda School of Public Health found water to be heart-protective as she looked at participants in the Adventist Health Study. She found that the women in the study who drank the most water were at the lowest risk of a fatal heart attack—a 40 percent lower risk, in fact, than those drinking the least amount of water. The men who drank the most water registered an even lower risk of fatal heart attack—a reduction of more than 50 percent![1] Dr. Chan discovered something even more shocking: You have to drink *water* to protect the heart. In the study, those participants who drank the most nonwater beverages, such as fruit juice, soda, coffee, and tea, *increased* their risk of a fatal heart attack. In fact, the study found that the women who drank the most non-water beverages increased their risk of a fatal heart attack two-and-a-half times; men in the same category increased their risk of a fatal heart attack by 50 percent.[2] So it's important to drink *water.*

Dr. Schroeder and his colleagues at Humboldt-University in Berlin found that drinking about two glasses of water and one-and-a-half ounces of mineral water daily kept blood pressure from dropping when healthy individuals stood up quickly.[3] Furthermore, Dr. Shannon at Vanderbilt University found two glasses of water to be effective treatment for orthostatic hypotension, a condition in which the nerves maintaining blood flow to the head when one stands up do not work properly.[4] It's important to drink sufficient water to prevent orthostatic hypotension. Dr. Eigenbrodt of the University of North Carolina has found that individuals with orthostatic hypotension have twice the risk of stroke compared with those whose blood pressure does not fall when standing from a reclining position.[5]

Here are some practical tips about drinking water:

♦ Drink large amounts (two to four eight-ounce glasses) of warm water in the morning to flush your digestive system and reduce the risk of constipation.

♦ Drink about ten or twelve eight-ounce glasses of water every day. As you begin exercising, especially if you do so in hot weather, it may be important to drink even more—at least three quarts a day to avoid constipation.

However, always follow your physician's instructions regarding fluid intake, as some individuals must restrict fluid intake because of heart or kidney failure.

◆ If possible, drink purified or distilled water, and drink water between meals. For optimal digestion of each meal, wait about an hour after a meal before drinking water and discontinue water intake about thirty minutes prior to meals.

If adopting a healthy lifestyle seems a difficult task, remember, your Creator, wants to help you take advantage of the health resources He has provided.

[1] J. Chan, "Water, Other Fluids, and Fatal Coronary Heart Disease," *American Journal of Epidemiology*, 2002, 155:827-833.

[2] Ibid.

[3] C. Schroeder, "Water Drinking Acutely Improves Orthostatic Tolerance in Healthy Subjects," *Circulation*, 2002, 106:2806.

[4] J. R. Shannon, "Drinking as a Treatment for Orthostatic Syndromes," *American Journal of Medicine*, April 1, 2002, 111 (5):355-360.

[5] M. L. Eigenbrodt, "Orthostatic Hypotension as a Risk Factor for Stroke: The Atherosclerosis Risk in Communities (ARIC) Study, 1987-1996," *Stroke*, vol. 31, 2000, pp. 2307-2313.

CHAPTER 5

Healing Emotions

Positive emotions have healing power. Therefore, it makes sense to cultivate cheerfulness, optimism, and hope.

Dr. Jonas and colleagues at the National Center for Health Statistics in Atlanta, Georgia, found that of those men and women studied, the most relaxed and cheerful also had the lowest risk of developing high blood pressure[1], a major risk factor for stroke[2] and coronary artery disease.[3] In the Atherosclerosis Risk in Communities (ARIC) Study, Dr. Williams and colleagues at the Centers for Disease Control and Prevention in Atlanta, Georgia, found that individuals less than sixty years old who had the lowest trait-anger scores had only one-third the risk of stoke compared to those with high trait-anger scores.[4] Remarkably, Dr. Williams found that anger and hostility increased the risk of stroke most for those persons who otherwise were at the lowest risk of heart- and blood vessel-related diseases.[5] In addition, Dr. Williams and colleagues discovered that individuals whose anger experiences were infrequent, brief, and of low intensity had less than half the risk of heart attack or death from coronary artery disease as did those with frequent, intense, and longer-lasting episodes of rage and fury.[6] Dr. Williams hypothesized that anger may induce blood vessel constriction, increase blood pressure, and increase the likelihood of blood clot formation, triggering rupture of cholesterol plaque in the artery wall with subsequent blood clot formation. Nearly every heart attack and the majority of strokes result from a blood clot that forms inside the artery, obstructing downstream blood flow.

Positive emotions actually help bring more blood to the heart muscle. In fact, Dr. Gullete and colleagues at Duke University Medical Center in North Carolina found that patients with coronary disease had only half the risk of reduced blood flow to their heart muscle during times of lowest tension, frustration, and sadness compared to times with high levels of these emotions.[7] Similarly, Dr. Kubzansky and colleagues at Harvard School of Public Health found that men who worried least about general world conditions, economic recession, or the future of the country had a 60-percent lower risk of nonfatal heart attack and about a 30-percent lower risk of all coronary disease as did men who worried most about these social conditions. In fact, Dr. Kubzansky found a dose-response relationship between social worry and coronary heart disease—the lower the social worry level, the lower the risk.[8]

Exercise may partially counteract the adverse effect of negative emotions on health. Dr. Blumenthal and colleagues at Duke University Medical Center in North Carolina studied heart attack patients who were depressed or who had little social support and found that among those who reported exercising regularly, the risk of another heart attack was nearly 30 percent lower than it was for those who did not report regular exercise.[9]

Optimism has also been found to promote health. Dr. Kubzansky and colleagues at Harvard University found optimistic men had better lung function and slower decline in lung function over time than did pessimistic men.[10] Additionally, Dr. Maruta and colleagues at Mayo Clinic in Minnesota found optimistic patients had a lower mortality risk over thirty years than did patients found to be pessimistic, using the optimism-pessimism scale of the Minnesota Multiphasic Personality Inventory (MMPI).[11] And Dr. Bowley and colleagues at the University of Plymouth, United Kingdom found optimistic patients able to return to their normal activities after a hernia operation more quickly than could patients with a pessimistic outlook. In fact, they found pessimism strongly correlated with a delayed return to normal activities.[12]

Optimism can even improve outcomes in cases of cancer. Dr. Levy and colleagues at the University of Pittsburgh School of Medicine found that those breast cancer survivors who were most optimistic were more likely to be alive after four years than were pessimistic patients.[13] Further, researchers at the University of California at Los Angeles surveyed 649 oncologists and found attitudes of hope and optimism to be the most significant factor in the successful treatment of more than 100,000 of their cancer patients.[14] Dr. Pert and her colleagues at the National Institute of Mental Health found monocytes (white blood cells) sensitive to neuropeptide chemicals produced and concentrated in the brain's limbic system—the center that controls emotions.[15]

Additionally, Dr. Byrnes and colleagues at the University of Miami in Florida observed greater activity of natural killer cells (white blood cells known to destroy cancer cells) among those women who were the most optimistic.[16] Dr. Segerstrom at the University of California at Los Angeles reported similar findings.[17]

Hope and optimism truly boost our cancer-fighting immune system. In fact, Dr. Kamen and Dr. Seligman and their colleagues at the University of Pennsylvania found optimistic adults had the strongest immune response, while pessimistic adults had weakest imune response among those studied.[18,19] Indeed, King Solomon's observation, "A merry heart doeth good like a medicine: but a broken spirit drieth the bones" (Proverbs 17:22), has a sound scientific basis. Start today to dismiss negative thoughts and foster a cheerful outlook.[20] Focus on your Creator and His goodness to you, and negative thoughts will begin to fade away.[21]

---

[1] B. S. Jonas, "Negative Affect as a Prospective Risk Factor for Hypertension," *Psychosomatic Medicine*, 2000; 62:188-196.

[2] N. M. Kaplan, *Kaplan's Clinical Hypertension*, eighth ed. (Philadelphia, Pa.: Lippincott Williams & Wilkins), © 2002, pp. 78.

[3] E. Braunwald, *Heart Disease: a Textbook of Cardiovascular Medicine*, sixth ed. (Philadelphia, Pa.: W. B. Saunders Co), © 2001, pp. 1050-1052.

[4] J. E. Williams, "The Association Between Trait Anger and Incident Stroke Risk: the Atherosclerosis Risk in Communities (ARIC) Study," *Stroke*, 2002; 33:13-20.

[5] Ibid.

[6] J. E. Williams, "Anger Proneness Predicts Coronary Heart Disease Risk:

Prospective Analysis From the Atherosclerosis Risk in Communities (ARIC) Study," *Circulation,* 2000; 101:2034-2039.

[7] A. R. Rozanski, "Impact of Psychological Factors on the Pathogenesis of Cardiovascular Disease and Implications for Therapy," *Circulation,* 1999; 99:2192-2217.

[8] L. D. Kubzansky, "Is Worrying Bad for Your Heart? A Prospective Study of Worry and Coronary Heart Disease in the Normative Aging Study," *Circulation,*1997; 95:818-824.

[9] J. A. Blumenthal, "Exercise, Depression, and Mortality After Myocardial Infarction in the ENRICHD Trial," *Med Sci Sports Exerc.,* May 2004; 36(5):746-55.

[10] L. D. Kubzansky, "Breathing Easy: a Prospective Study of Optimism and Pulmonary Function in the Normative Aging Study," *Annals of Behavioral Medicine,* Fall 2002; 24(4):345-53.

[11] T. Maruta, "Optimists vs. Pessimists: Survival Rate Among Medical Patients Over a 30-Year Period," *Mayo Clin Proc.,* February 2000; 75(2):140-3.

[12] D. M. Bowley, "Dispositional Pessimism Predicts Delayed Return to Normal Activities After Inguinal Hernia Operation," *Surgery,* February 2003; 133(2):141-6.

[13] S. M. Levy, "Survival Hazards Analysis in First Recurrent Breast Cancer Patients: Seven-Year Follow-up," *Psychosomatic Medicine,* September-October 1988; 50(5):520-8.

[14] B. Q. Hafen, *Mind/Body Health: the Effects of Attitudes, Emotions, and Relationships,* Boston, Ma.: Allyn and Bacon), © 1996, p. 513.

[15] Ibid., p. 515.

[16] D. M. Byrnes, "Stressful Events, Pessimism, Natural Killer Cell Cytotoxicity, and Cytotoxic/Suppressor T Cells in HIV+ Black Women at Risk for Cervical Cancer," *Psychosomatic Medicine,* November-December 1998; 60(6):714-22.

[17] S. C. Segerstrom, "Optimism Is Associated With Mood, Coping, and Immune Change in Response to Stress," *J Pers Soc Psychology,* June 1998; 74(6):1646-55.

[18] B. Q. Hafen, *Mind/Body Health: the Effects of Attitudes, Emotions, and Relationships,* Boston, Ma.: Allyn and Bacon), © 1996, p. 513.

[19] M. E. Seligman, "Explanatory Style and Cell-Mediated Immunity in Elderly Men and Women," *Health Psychology,* 1991; 10(4):229-35.

[20] E. G. White, *The Ministry of Healing,* (Nampa, Id.: Pacific Press Publishing Association), p. 251.

[21] See 2 Corinthians 3:18; 10:4, 5.

CHAPTER 6

Vegetables Protect Health

Before we have a need, the Creator is working to supply that need. After Adam and Eve sinned, the environment became harsh—even toxic. It is even more so today. The Lord knew this would be the case, so He commanded Adam to "eat the herb of the field" (Genesis 3:18) for added protection. Today the scientific literature is full of evidence showing that produce—vegetables—protects our health. Dr. Joshipura and his colleagues at the Harvard School of Public Health found that those Americans eating the most fruits and vegetables are at a 20 percent lower risk of coronary heart disease than those eating the least produce. Furthermore, Dr. Joshipura found a 23 percent decrease in coronary disease for every one serving increase in green leafy vegetables. Vitamin C-rich fruits and vegetables were also very protective against devastating coronary disease. His study also showed those eating the most fruit and vegetables were at a 31 percent lower risk of stroke.[1]

Likewise, Dr. Cohen at the Fred Hutchinson Cancer Research Center in Seattle, Washington, found that men eating three or more servings per week of cruciferous vegetables (broccoli, cauliflower, kale, Brussels sprouts, et cetera) were at a 41 percent lower risk of prostate cancer than were men eating the fewest servings of cruciferous vegetables.[2] Furthermore, Dr. Potter of the American Institute for Cancer Research in Washington, D.C., has stated that at least 20 percent of all cancers could be prevented if Americans ate five servings daily of fruits and vegetables.[3] Cancers most likely to be prevented by generous intake of garden and orchard produce are those of the mouth, throat, esophagus, lung, stomach, colon, rectum, voice box, pancreas, breast, and bladder.

In order to receive optimal protection from produce consider these recommendations:

◆ Eat nine half-cup servings of fruits and vegetables each day.

◆ Enjoy one to three half-cup servings of dark green, leafy vegetables daily as part of your nine total servings.

◆ As part of your daily produce intake, increase intake of vitamin C-rich fruits and vegetables (bell peppers, Brussels sprouts, pink grapefruit, kiwi, oranges).

◆ Maximize intake of yellow and orange vegetables and fruits (sweet potatoes, apricots, etc.), which are rich in carotene pigments. This will increase the removal of toxic free radicals from body tissues and prevent a source of cholesterol buildup in arterial walls as well as injury to DNA that can lead to cancer.

Also, focus your attention on fruits and vegetables with the highest antioxidant content (blueberries, strawberries, kale, spinach, garlic). Furthermore, be aware that pesticide residues and chemical coatings may contaminate some fresh produce. Therefore, I recommend peeling the following items (or washing them with mild edible soap): apples, bell peppers, cucumbers, green beans, peaches, pears, spinach, strawberries, tomatoes, winter squash, and plums.

The more you consider the powerful benefits of fruits and vegetables, the more you understand the truth of these words, "But my God shall supply all your need according to his riches in glory" (Philippians 4:19).

---

[1] K. J. Joshipura, "The Effect of Fruit and Vegetable Intake on Risk for Coronary Heart Disease," *Annual of Internal Medicine*, 2001, 134:1106-1114.

[2] J. H. Cohen, "Fruit and Vegetable Intakes and Prostate Cancer Risk," *Journal of the National Cancer Institute*, vol. 92, no. 1, pp. 61-68.

[3] J. D. Potter, "Executive Summary of Food Nutrition and the Prevention of Cancer: a Global Perspective," American Institute for Cancer Research, 1997.

CHAPTER 7

Choose Carbohydrates

Many Americans are avoiding carbohydrates. Others are asking, "Are carbohydrates a friend or enemy?" There's an old saying, "If all else fails, read the owner's manual." Let's look at the carbohydrate content of the diet that received the Creator's highest endorsement. He called it "very good" (Genesis 1:31).

The average carbohydrate content of 195 fruits, vegetables, grains, and beans is 78 percent. Now add nuts and seeds. The average carbohydrate content of 227 fruits, grains, beans, vegetables, nuts, and seeds is 60 percent. And the protein content is 14 percent.[1] So we see that in the Creator's diet, the carbohydrate content drops no lower than 60 percent even if we give nuts an equal weight with other categories of food, which I don't recommend, since nuts and seeds are best used as condiments.[2] If you use them as condiments, then the carbohydrate content of the Creator's diet becomes 65 percent to 70 percent.

Why did the Creator load His food for the human family with carbohydrates? Carbohydrates help raise brain serotonin, which may help lower risk of depression and optimize thyroid function, making it easier to stay trim. Carbohydrates are used in the manufacture of special proteins and fats on body cells. These proteins and fats have special sugars attached to them, which are needed for cells to communicate with each other. Only carbohydrate fuel maximizes physical endurance.[3] Carbohydrates are also packaged alongside vital protective nutrients—flavanoids, phytochemicals, and antioxidants. Finally, the fuel of choice for the brain is glucose, which is primarily made from carbohydrate!

Beyond missing these carbohydrate benefits, are there other problems with low-carbohydrate/high-protein diets? Yes. Such diets leech calcium from bones.[4] They increase workload of the kidneys[5] and are about half as effective as a high- carbohydrate, high-fiber diet at lowering cholesterol.[6] They increase urine calcium, which may increase risk of kidney stones. Low-carbohydrate diets change body physiology to that of a starvation state.[7]

Have medical researchers found low-carbohydrate diets safe and effective? Dr. Bravata and colleagues at Stanford University reviewed 107 studies of 94 low-carbohydrate diets between 1966 and 2003 and found that among patients carrying excessive weight, the weight loss was not due to carbohydrate restriction. Weight loss was due to diet duration and calorie restriction. Furthermore, low-carbohydrate diets did not lower cholesterol, triglycerides, blood sugar, fasting insulin, or blood pressure. Finally, the lowest carbohydrate diets were studied in only 71 people. Summarizing her review of the low-carbohydrate diet, Dr. Bravata states, "We know little of its effects or consequences."[8]

Our Creator originally provided a diet rich in carbohydrates. When choosing this very best diet, your health will flourish.

[1] Food Processor for Windows, version 7.81, ESHA Research, Salem, Ore., © 2001.

[2] See E. G. White, *Counsels on Diets and Foods,* pp. 273, 274.

[3] M. Fogelholm, "Dairy Products, Meat, and Sports Performance," *Sports Medicine,* 2003, 33 (8):615-631.

[4] L. K. Massey, "Dietary Animal and Plant Protein and Human Bone Health: A Whole Foods Approach," *Journal of Nutrition,* March 2003, 133 (3):862S-865S. J. Eisenstein, "High-Protein Weight-Loss Diets: Are They Safe and Do They Work? A Review of the Experimental and Epidemiologic Data," *Nutrition Review,* July 2002, 60 (7 Pt 1):189-200.

[5] A. R. Skov, "Changes in Renal Function During Weight Loss Induced By High vs Low-Protein Low-Fat Diets in Overweight Subjects," *International Journal of Obesity Related Metabolic Disorders,* November 1999, 23 (11):1170-1177.

[6] K. O'Dea, "The Effects of Diet Differing in Fat, Carbohydrate, and Fiber on Carbohydrate and Lipid Metabolism in Type II Diabetes," *Journal of the American Dietetic Association,* August 1989, 89 (8):1076-1086.

[7] D. M. Bravata, "Efficacy and Safety of Low-Carbohydrate Diets: A Systematic Review," *Journal of the American Medical Association,* 2003, 289:1837-1850.

[8] Ibid.

CHAPTER 8

Eat Nuts and Seeds Daily

Part of the Creator's original diet was nuts. Recent scientific literature confirms the wisdom of including this nutrient-dense food in your diet.

Dr. Jiang at Harvard Medical School found that women eating nuts five or more times a week were at a 27 percent lower risk of type 2 diabetes than were those eating them never or almost never. Also, he found women eating the most nuts gained the least weight over 16 years compared with those eating nuts less frequently.[1]

Over a period of seventeen years, Dr. Albert at Brigham and Women's Hospital in Boston found that men eating nuts two or more times a week were at half the risk of sudden death compared with men who rarely or never ate nuts.[2]

Dr. Hu, of the Harvard School of Public Health, found that women eating one handful of nuts more than five times a week were at less than half the risk of coronary artery disease as were women who rarely or never ate nuts.[3]

Nuts are rich in vitamin E, magnesium, and monounsaturated fat, all of which are believed to reduce the risk of heart disease and diabetes or its complications.

Nuts and other plant foods contain good fats. However, the food industry has taken plant fat and converted it into one of the most harmful of all foods—trans fat, commonly known as "partially hydrogenated vegetable oil."

Dr. Salmeron at the Harvard School of Public Health estimated that 40 percent of type 2 diabetes could be eliminated if we replaced partially hydrogenated vegetable oil with nonhydrogenated oil. In fact, every 2 percent increase in the number of calories from trans fat raises the risk of type 2 diabetes by 39 percent.[4] Additionally, Dr. Morris at the Rush Institute for Healthy Aging in Chicago, found that eating significant amounts of "partially hydrogenated" vegetable oil increased one's risk of Alzheimer's disease by nearly two-and-a-half times.[5]

Therefore, avoid all packaged foods that contain partially hydrogenated vegetable oil, *but* by all means eat one ounce—about a cupped handful—of unsalted nuts daily. Excellent choices are almonds, English walnuts, hazelnuts, and pecans. Also, daily eat two to three tablespoons of one of the following seeds:

◆ Sesame seeds (calcium, copper, and iron).
◆ Pumpkin seeds (iron, magnesium, L-arginine, and zinc).
◆ Sunflower seeds (copper, magnesium, Vitamin E, and selenium).
◆ Watermelon seeds (zinc and magnesium).

---

[1] R. Jiang, "Nut and Peanut Butter Consumption and Risk of Type 2 Diabetes in Women," *Journal of the American Medical Association,* November 2002, 288 (20):2554-2560.

[2] C. M. Albert, "Nut Consumption and Decreased Risk of Sudden Cardiac Death in the Physicians' Health Study," *Archives of Internal Medicine*, 2002, 162:1382-1387.

[3] F. B. Hu, "Frequent Nut Consumption and Risk of Coronary Heart Disease in Women: Prospective Cohort Study," *BMJ*, 1998, 317:1341-1345.

[4] J. Salmeron, "Dietary Fat Intake and Risk of Type 2 Diabetes in Women," *American Journal of Clinical Nutrition*, 2001, 73:1019-1026.

[5] M. C. Morris, "Dietary Fats and the Risk of Incident Alzheimer Disease," *Archives of Neurology*, February 2003, 60 (2):194-200.

CHAPTER 9

Whole Grains Are the Best

God is interested in you. He wants you to have better nutrition than you may have settled for in the past. Let's look at an important part of the Creator's diet for human beings—whole grains.

Notice how protective whole grains are. Dr. Montonen at the National Public Health Institute in Helsinki, Finland has found that those eating the most whole grains are at a 61 percent lower risk of developing type 2 diabetes than are those eating the fewest whole grains and that the more you eat whole grains in place of refined grains, the lower your risk.[1] Similarly, Dr. Fung from Simmons College in Boston demonstrated that men with the greatest intake of whole grains are at a 30 percent lower risk of type 2 diabetes than are those eating the fewest whole grains. Interestingly enough, she also found that those men eating the largest amount of *refined* grains did not increase their risk of type 2 diabetes.[2] In other words, to lower risk of type 2 diabetes, it is not enough to avoid white rice and "enriched" wheat flour or white bread, you have to eat whole grains.

In addition, Dr. Liu and colleagues at Harvard's School of Public Health in Boston have found that women eating the most whole grains were at a 25 percent lower risk of coronary artery disease.[3] Dr. Liu and his colleagues have also shown that women eating the most whole grains had the lowest risk of stroke—a 31 percent decrease.[4] Other health-related factors were controlled for in these studies, thus the results indicated may be attributed to the effect of whole grains. The evidence seems clear—the more you choose to eat whole grains in place of refined grains, the lower your risk of diabetes, heart disease, and stroke.

Choosing whole grains will also help you maximize your fiber intake, which may help lower risk of colon cancer. After a combined analysis of thirteen case-control studies, Dr. Howe at the University of Toronto determined that those individuals eating the most fiber were at a 47 percent lower risk of colon cancer than those consuming low amounts of fiber.[5]

Here are some of the reasons our Creator put fiber in whole grains:

◆ Fiber in whole grains helps remove cholesterol from the intestine so that it is not reabsorbed back into the blood stream.

◆ It holds water, rendering the stool large and soft.

◆ It reduces pressure inside the bowel, which lowers risk of multiple common bowel diseases, such as diverticulitis.

◆ Whole grains are fermented by colon bacteria, generating bowel-nourishing and colon cancer-preventing short-chain fatty acids, and hindering growth of harmful bacteria, while supporting growth of beneficial bacteria.

To enjoy all these benefits and many more:

◆ Eat six or more half-cup servings daily of 100 percent whole grains.

◆ Choose brown rice instead of white.

◆ Eat whole-wheat (brown) pasta in place of semolina (tan) pasta. If you have type 2 diabetes or want to lose weight, use even whole wheat pasta sparingly.

◆ Use 100 percent whole-wheat bread with no "enriched" wheat flour in the list of ingredients.

◆ Choose breakfast cereals made only from whole grain.

◆ Use whole-wheat flour or whole wheat pastry flour in recipes, rather than white flour, if at all possible.

At Lifestyle Center of America, physicians have noticed that blood sugar rises sharply when patients with diabetes eat even small amounts of white or "enriched" wheat flour. If you want optimal health, always choose the whole package the Creator provided. Optimal health depends upon every part of the whole grain.

[1] J. Montonen, "Whole-Grain and Fiber Intake and the Incidence of Type 2 Diabetes," *American Journal of Clinical Nutrition*, 2003, 77:622-629.

[2] T. T. Fung, "Whole-Grain Intake and The risk of Type 2 Diabetes: A Prospective Study in Men," *American Journal of Clinical Nutrition*, 2002, 76:535-540.

[3] S. Liu, "Whole-Grain Consumption and Risk of Coronary Heart Disease: Results From the Nurses' Health Study," *American Journal of Clinical Nutrition*, 1999, 70:412-419.

[4] S. Liu, "Whole Grain Consumption and Risk of Ischemic Stroke in Women: A Prospective Study," *Journal of the American Medical Association*, 2000, 284:1534-1540.

[5] G. R. Howe, "Dietary Intake of Fiber and Decreased Risk of Cancers of the Colon and Rectum: Evidence From the Combined Analysis of 13 Case-Control Studies," *Journal of the National Cancer Institute*, December 16, 1992, 84 (24):1887-1896.

CHAPTER 10

Flaxseed Is Good for You

Our Creator is attentive to and interested in the smallest details of our lives. Flaxseed is an example of something small with powerful benefits. Flaxseed is rich in a fat—alpha-linolenic acid—that is essential to health and which the body cannot manufacture. This essential fat reduces inflammation[1] in the body, helps prevent blood clots that cause heart attack and stroke,[2] helps protect against deadly heart rhythms,[3] lowers cholesterol and triglycerides,[4] and helps arteries open wider.[5] These essential fats have improved coronary heart disease, high blood pressure, type 2 diabetes, kidney disease, rheumatoid arthritis, ulcerative colitis, Crohn's disease, and chronic obstructive lung disease.[6] Essential fats are critical for proper brain development and function and are needed to make hormones, called thromboxanes, leukotrienes, and prostaglandins which help lower blood pressure, prevent blood clots, keep arteries open, optimize immune function, and lower inflammation.[7]

Dr. Hu and colleagues at Harvard Medical School found that those individuals with the greatest intake of alpha-linolenic acid were at nearly *half* the risk of a fatal heart attack compared to those eating the least alpha-linolenic acid.[8]

Furthermore, Dr. de Lorgeril and colleagues reported in the *The Lancet* that when patients who experienced a heart attack were placed on a diet high in alpha-linolenic acid, their risk of dying was 70 percent lower after five years than for those eating the standard post-heart attack prudent diet.[9]

Eating fish brings similar benefits. However, along with the protective essential fats found in fish are toxins such as PCBs, DDT, DDE, and heavy metals, such as mercury. In fact, Dr. Guallar and colleagues at Johns Hopkins School of Public Health found high mercury level in body tissues can result in more than twice the normal risk of heart attack. And Dr. Schober at the National Center for Health Statistics found mercury levels to be four times higher in women who had eaten three or more servings of fish during the previous month compared to women who had eaten no fish during that same period. Clearly we become what we eat. If our food contains toxic chemicals, so will our tissues. Therefore, it is best to obtain vital essential fats from plant sources. Follow these guidelines:

- Replace meat, fish, milk, eggs, and cheese with vegetables, beans, whole grains, fruits, nuts, and seeds.
- Daily eat one to two tablespoons of whole flaxseed, freshly ground.
- Eat one ounce of English walnuts three times a week.
- Severely limit visible fats and processed oils, which can reduce production of vital essential fats.
- Increase intake of foods rich in monounsatured fat, such as olives, avocado, hazelnuts, almonds, peanuts, and pecans.

God designed and created our bodies. Thus, He knows best how we can achieve optimal health, partly by paying attention to little things with powerful health-promoting benefits—like flaxseed.

[1] L. S. Rallidis, "Dietary Alpha-Linolenic Acid Decreases C-Reactive Protein, Serum Amyloid A, and Interleukin-6 in Dyslipidaemic Patients," *Atherosclerosis*, April 2003, 167 (2):237-242.

[2] D. Lanzmann-Petithory, "Alpha-Linolenic Acid and Cardiovascular Diseases," *Journal of Nutrtional, Health, and Aging*, 2001 5 (3):179-183.

[3] B. Davis, "Essential Fatty Acids in Vegetarian Nutrition," Vegetarian Nutrition: a Dietetic Practice Group of The American Dietetic Association, Andrews University Nutrition Department, 2002.

[4] D. R. Illingworth, "The Influence of Dietary N-3 Fatty Acids on Plasma Lipids and Lipoproteins," *Annual of the New York Academy of Science*, 1993, 676:70-82.

[5] B. Davis, "Essential Fatty Acids in Vegetarian Nutrition," Vegetarian Nutrition: a Dietetic Practice Group of The American Dietetic Association, Andrews University Nutrition Department, 2002.

[6] A. P. Simopoulos, "Essential Fatty Acids in Health and Chronic Disease," *American Journal of Clinical Nutrition*, 1999, 70 (suppl):560S-569S.

[7] B. Davis, "Essential Fatty Acids in Vegetarian Nutrition," Vegetarian Nutrition: a Dietetic Practice Group of The American Dietetic Association, Andrews University Nutrition Department, 2002.

[8] F. B. Hu, "Dietary Intake of Alpha-Linolenic Acid and Risk of Fatal Ischemic Heart Disease Among Women."

[9] M. De Lorgeril, "Mediterranean Alpha-Linolenic Acid-Rich Diet in Secondary Prevention of Coronary Heart Disease," *The Lancet*, June 11, 1994, 343 (8911):1454-1459.

CHAPTER 11

Choose Carob Instead of Chocolate

Chocolate can cause a variety of unhealthful conditions in the body. Consider choosing carob over chocolate to avoid chocolate's adverse effects on your health.

Doctors Wright and Castell reported in the *American Journal of Digestive Diseases* that pressure in the muscle that helps keep acid from entering the esophagus dropped nearly 50 percent after participants drank only four ounces of chocolate syrup.[1]

In one study, Dr. Minton and colleagues found that 83 percent of women with painful, tender, palpable, breast nodules of fibrocystic breast disease had complete resolution of these nodules within one to six months of eliminating coffee, tea, colas, and chocolate from their diets.[2] These drinks contain caffeine and/or theobromine, methylxanthines known to rev up cell activity to an abnormal level.

Dr. Nguyen and colleagues reported in the journal *Hormone and Metabolism Research* that a single three-and-a-half ounce dark chocolate bar increased calcium loss in the urine by 147 percent and oxalate by 213 percent compared to the calcium loss experienced by those eating the same amount of sugar but without ingesting chocolate.[3] The most commonly occurring kidney stone is made of calcium oxalate. Thus, chocolate may increase risk of kidney stones and increase loss of calcium from bones.

The following are other reasons to choose carob over chocolate:

◆ Large amounts of sugar are needed to cover chocolate's bitter taste.

◆ It is "calorie dense" with more than 250 calories in three-and-a-half ounces.

◆ It contains caffeine.

◆ It contains more theobromine than it does caffeine.

◆ It contains brain-altering chemicals such as anandamides, stronger cousins of which are found in marijuana.[4]

◆ It contains addiction-promoting components such as phenylethylamine,[5] which is related to amphetamine.

◆ Chocolate upsets appetite control[6] and is high in fat, having 50 percent or more of its calories coming from fat.

◆ Chocolate contains tryptamine,[7] known to disrupt serotonin metabolism.[8]

Thus, chocolate is bitter in more ways than one. The Creator's chosen foods do not need lots of added sugar to make them appetizing. Switching from chocolate to carob or to fresh fruits, such as apples, pears, peaches, plums, cherries, apricots, and berries, will help you improve your health and give you a clearer mind.

---

[1] L. E. Wright, "The Adverse Effect of Chocolate on Lower Esophageal Sphincter Pressure," *American Journal of Digestive Diseases*, August 1975, 20 (8):703-707.

[2] J. P. Minton, "Clinical and Biochemical Studies on Methylxanthine-Related Fibrocystic Breast Disease," *Surgery,* August 1981, 90 (2):299-304.

[3] N. U. Nguyen, "Increase in Calciuria and Oxaluria After a Single Chocolate Bar Load," *Hormone Metabolism Research,* August 1994, 26 (8):383-386.

[4] J. S. James, "Marijuana and chocolate," *AIDS Treatment News,* October 18, 1996, (No 257):3, 4. E. Di Tomaso "Brain Cannabinoids in Chocolate," *Nature,* August 22, 1996, 382 (6593):677-678.

[5] G. Ziegleder, "Occurrence of Beta-Phenylethylamine and Its Derivatives in Cocoa and Cocoa Products," *Z Lebensm Unters Forsch,* September 1992, 195 (3):235-238.

[6] T. Tuomisto, "Psychological and Physiological Characteristics of Sweet Food 'Addiction,' " *International Journal of Eating Disorders,* March 25, 1999, (2):169-175.

[7] T. Herraiz, "Tetrahydro-Beta-Carbolines, Potential Neuroactive Alkaloids, in Chocolate and Cocoa," *Journal of Agricultural Food Chemistry,* October 2000 48 (10):4900-4904.

[8] B. E. Baldwin, "Problems With Chocolate," *The Journal of Health and Healing,* 2002, 24 (3):3-6, 11, 15.

CHAPTER 12

Avoid Caffeine and Refined Sugar

There are a growing list of reasons today to leave caffeine and refined sugar out of your beverages. Here are a few of them.

Dr. Ludwig of Children's Hospital in Boston found the risk of childhood obesity increased 60 percent for each additional serving of sugar-sweetened drink.[1]

Excessive weight gain in childhood fuels development of type 2 diabetes in children.[2]

Dr. Slattery of the University of Utah found those individuals who consumed the most table sugar were at 59 percent greater risk of colon cancer than those consuming modest amounts. Additionally, he found that those who ate the most table sugar *and* who were sedentary, excessively overweight, and ate little dietary fiber were at a risk for colon cancer more than four-and-a-half times greater than those who did not have these factors in their lives.[3]

Two soft drinks contain twenty teaspoons of sugar, and the average American drinks more than 560 twelve-ounce cans of soft drinks every year! In fact, the average sugar intake for Americans is more than thirty teaspoons per day! Yet, Dr. Kijak of Loma Linda University has demonstrated that after twenty-four teaspoons of sugar, the number of bacteria destroyed by white blood cells dropped from fourteen to one.[4] No wonder we need antibiotics so often! It's important to note that we also depend on these sugar-hindered white blood cells to protect us from viruses and cancer.

Refined sugar has been shown to cause low blood sugar, reduced physical endurance in athletes, and reduced mental vigor in students.

Leaving off caffeine will also benefit health.

Dr. Graham at the University of Guelph in Canada found that ingesting caffeine before an Oral Glucose Tolerance test caused insulin levels to be 37 percent higher. Yet, despite higher insulin levels, blood sugar rose 24 percent during the test.[5] Thus, caffeine forces the pancreas to pour out more insulin, but also worsens insulin resistance, leaving blood sugar higher. Caffeine worsens diabetes and pushes human physiology toward a diabetic state.

Studies have also shown that caffeine contributes to a host of health problems. For example, it increases blood pressure, stress hormone levels in the blood, pressure in the eyes, arterial stiffness, calcium loss from the kidneys, risk of spontaneous abortion, stomach acid, and coronary artery wall resistance. Caffeine also *reduces* coronary blood flow reserves and blood flow in the optic nerve and the retina. As well, it may precipitate abnormal heart rhythms, induce seizures in those with seizure disorders, contribute to fibrocystic breast disease, and worsen premenstrual syndrome. And Dr. Corti at the University Hospital in Zurich,

Switzerland found that decaffeinated coffee raised blood pressure and increased sympathetic nervous system activity in muscles about as much as regular coffee.[6]

Dr. Palmer and colleagues at the Boston University School of Medicine found that the risk of heart attack increased for those drinking five or more cups of coffee daily regardless of whether they were smokers or not, and that those drinking the most coffee had a risk of heart attack two-and-a-half times greater than those drinking minimal amounts of coffee.[7]

If you have an addictive relationship with a food or beverage, the best thing to do is leave it off for good. When thirsty, choose the beverage the Creator provided to quench our thirst—pure water.

---

[1] D. S. Ludwig, "Relation Between Consumption of Sugar-Sweetened Drinks and Childhood Obesity: A Prospective, Observational Analysis," *The Lancet*, February 17, 2001, 357 (9255):505-508.

[2] S. Ranjana, "Prevalence of Impaired Glucose Tolerance among Children and Adolescents with Marked Obesity," *New England Journal of Medicine*, 2002, 346:802-810.

[3] M. L. Slattery, "Dietary Sugar and Colon Cancer," Cancer Epidemiological Biomarkers Preview, September 6, 1997, (9):677-685.

[4] E. Kijak, "Relationship of Blood Sugar Level and Leukocytic Phagocytosis," Southern California Dental Association, 1964, 32 (9):349-351.

[5] T. E. Graham, "Caffeine Ingestion Elevates Plasma Insulin Response in Humans During an Oral Glucose Tolerance Test," *Canadian Journal of Physiology and Pharmacology*, July 2001, 79 (7):559-565.

[6] R. Corti, "Coffee Acutely Increases Sympathetic Nerve Activity and Blood Pressure Independently of Caffeine Content," *Circulation*, 2002, 106:2935.

[7] J. R. Palmer, "Coffee Consumption and Myocardial Infarction in Women," *American Journal of Epidemiology*, April 15, 1995, 141 (8):724-731.

CHAPTER 13

Don't Forget Vitamin B$_{12}$

He was one of my favorite patients at Lifestyle Center of America. He had been a lifestyle educator and a vegetarian for many years. The last two years, he had became a total vegetarian, eating only whole grains, beans, fruits, vegetables, nuts, and seeds. However, this patient, who knew so much about health, had a potentially serious problem. He had an elevated level of an amino acid called homocysteine. Also, this patient had a very low vitamin B$_{12}$ level— at the very bottom of the range.

Why was this important? Researchers have discovered if blood levels of this amino acid—homocysteine—are high, it can lead to damage of arteries and brain tissue, probably through "oxidation," a process that occurs when free radicals, a dangerous type of oxygen, are released by our body cells and chemically damage surrounding tissue, including arteries, cholesterol, and DNA. If the level of homocysteine is high, more tissue damage from "free radicals" may occur. So if you want optimal blood vessel and brain health, keep your level of homocysteine low by eating plenty of vitamin B$_{12}$. A relative had been total vegetarian for nearly forty years. Other than eating a small amount of egg in an ocassional entreé, this individual was a total vegetarian. At eighty years of age, this person still enjoyed good health. He was not on medications, did not have high blood pressure, and had never been in the hospital. He had no cancer or heart disease. However, after turning eighty, this person began losing memory function. He also developed difficulty walking and getting out of a chair. Signs of Parkinson's disease and dementia became noticeable.

Why would one who followed such a healthy diet have these symptoms? What was the problem? Then we measured his blood homocysteine level. It was over twice the upper limit of normal. This individual did not take vitamin B$_{12}$ all the years he had been a total vegetarian. Medical research has shown that individuals with high levels of the amino acid homocysteine have a two or three times greater risk of dying of a heart attack or a stroke as do individuals with lower blood levels of this amino acid.[1]

Additionally, individuals with the highest homocysteine levels have been found to be at more than four times greater risk of Alzheimer's disease.[2] Thus, it is important to keep this amino acid low. In order to do this you must get an adequate amount of vitamin B$_{12}$. As you move to a plant-based diet, it is very important to get extra vitamin B$_{12}$.[3] I recommend chewing a vitamin B$_{12}$ supplement—at least 500 micrograms—daily. Not most days, but every day! Taking 500mcg of vitamin B$_{12}$ daily is probably the minimum needed to keep homocysteine at an acceptable level for most people following a total vegetarian diet. This is because only about 1 percent of the 500mcg of vitamin B_{12} is absorbed, and the current daily value for vitamin B_{12} is six micrograms.[4]

I also recommend generous amounts of two other B vitamins, namely folic acid and pyridoxine, or vitamin B_6. Eat plenty of foods rich in folic acid—such as beans, dark green leafy vegetables, and citrus fruits. Sesame seeds, garbanzo beans, flaxseed, pistachio nuts, as well as garlic and bananas, are rich in vitamin B_6. These three B vitamins—B_{12}, folic acid, and B_6—can help lower your homocysteine level. Thus, as you transition to a plant-based diet, reach out daily and take that tiny vitamin B_{12} tablet. You'll be glad you did! Remember, chew it, and don't take it at the same meal as a multivitamin, because the minerals in the multivitamin may render vitamin B_{12} inactive.[5]

---

[1] S. E. Vollset, "Plasma Total Homocysteine and Cardiovascular and Noncardiovascular Mortality: The Hordaland Homocysteine Study," *American Journal of Clinical Nutrition*, 2001,74:130-136.

[2] R. Clarke, "Folate, Vitamin B_{12}, and Serum Total Homocysteine Levels in Confirmed Alzheimer Disease," *Archives of Neurology*, November 1998, 55 (11):1449-1455.

[3] W. Herrmann, "Vitamin B-12 Status, Particularly Holotranscobalamin II and Methylmalonic Acid Concentrations, and Hyperhomocysteinemia in Vegetarians," *American Journal of Clinical Nutrition*, 2003, 78:131-136.

[4] Food and Nutrition Board, Institute of Medicine, "Dietary Reference Intakes for Thiamin, Riboflavin, Niacin, Vitamin B_6, Folate, Vitamin B_{12}, Pantothenic Acid, Biotin, and Choline," Washington, D. C.: National Academy Press, 2000, p. 308.

[5] S. J. Christensen, Weimar Institute's *NEWSTART® Lifestyle Cookbook* (Nashville, Tenn.: Thomas Nelson Publishers), p. 192.

CHAPTER 14

The Benefits of Sunlight and Vitamin D

Our Creator wants us to enjoy good health (see 3 John 2). Many, however, are missing the mighty benefits of sunshine, because most of us spend nearly all our time indoors. According to Dr. Michael Holick, an expert in vitamin D physiology from Boston University, vitamin D greatly increases the ability of the intestines to absorb calcium and phosphorus, helping to prevent osteoporosis, osteomalacia, fibromyalgia, muscle weakness, hypertension, and rickets.[1]

Vitamin D also modulates the immune system, helping to prevent the dysfunctional immune system seen in such autoimmune diseases as type 1 diabetes and systemic lupus.[2] Importantly, vitamin D slows the rate of cell division and influences cells to fully mature, thus, helping to prevent cancer of the colon, prostate, breast, and ovary.[3]

More than a decade ago, researchers in Lyon, France reported that 1,200 mg. of elemental calcium plus 800 IU of vitamin D reduced the risk of hip fracture 43 percent over a period of eighteen months in healthy women aged seventy-eight to ninety years. Bone density increased by nearly 3 percent, whereas bone density in the placebo group dropped nearly 5 percent in that time period.[4]

Studies at the Institute of Child Health in London found that Finnish children given vitamin D had an 88 percent lower risk of type 1 diabetes than those not given vitamin D. In addition, children who regularly took the Finnish recommended dose of vitamin D (2,000 IU) had a 78 percent lower risk of type 1 diabetes than children who took less than 2,000 IU a day.[5]

If you are struggling with osteoporosis, fibromyalgia, high blood pressure, muscle weakness, systemic lupus, or if you want to lower your risk of cancer—especially if you spend most of your time indoors or have darker skin—take vitamin D seriously. At Lifestyle Center of America we check the 25-hydroxyvitamin D level on every patient. I recommend the following guidelines regarding vitamin D to my patients:

- Keep your vitamin D (25-hydroxyvitamin D) level between 40-60ng/ml.
- Get approximately fifteen minutes of exposure to direct sunlight on your face, hands, and arms at least three times a week. Be careful never to burn your skin or get so much sunlight exposure that your skin turns pink, as excessive exposure to sunlight can lead to skin cancer and may increase your risk of melanoma. You don't even need to tan your skin to get all the vitamin D you need.
- Remember that adequate vitamin D protection requires exposure to sunlight for only one-fourth of the time that

is required to burn the skin. Be very careful not to get too much sunlight exposure!

We were made to be in the sun. If you can't get out in the sunshine for about fifteen minutes each day, consider taking a vitamin D supplement, but never exceed a daily total of 2,000 IU, the maximum considered safe by the National Academy of Sciences.[6]

[1] M. F. Holick, "Vitamin D and Bone Health," *Journal of Nutrition*, April, 1996, 126 (4 Suppl):1159S-1164S. "Vitamin D: A Millennium Perspective," *Journal of Cellular Biochemistry*, 2003, 88:296-307.

[2] H. F. Deluca, "Vitamin D: Its Role and Uses in Immunology," FASEB J, 2001, 15:2579-2585. M. F. Holick, "Vitamin D: A Millennium Perspective," *Journal of Cellular Biochemistry*, 2003, 88:296-307.

[3] M. F. Holick, "Vitamin D: A Millennium Perspective," *Journal of Cellular Biochemistry*, 2003, 88:296-307. D. M. Freedman, "Sunlight and Mortality From Breast, Ovarian, Colon, Prostate, and Non-Melanoma Skin Cancer: A Composite Death Certificate Based Case-Control Study," *Occupational Environmental Medicine*, 2002, 59:257-262. C. F. Garland,"Serum 25-Hydroxyvitamin D and Colon Cancer: Eight-Year Prospective Study," *The Lancet*, January 13, 1990, 335 (8681):1176-1178.

[4] M. C. Chapuy, "Vitamin D3 and Calcium to Prevent Hip Fractures in the Elderly Women," *New England Journal of Medicine*, December 3, 1992, 327 (23):1637-1642.

[5] E. Hypponen, "Intake of Vitamin D and Risk of Type 1 Diabetes: A Birth-Cohort Study," *The Lancet*, November 3, 2001, 358 (9292):1500-1503.

[6] V. R. Young, Chair, Standing Committee on the Scientific Evaluation of Dietary Reference Intakes, Food and Nutrition Board, Institute of Medicine. *Dietary Reference Intakes for Calcium, Phosphorus, Magnesium, Vitamin D, and Fluoride* (Washington, D. C.: National Academy Press, 1997).

CHAPTER 15

Eat Plants to Avoid Disease

On December 23, 2003, the U.S. Department of Agriculture made a preliminary diagnosis of Mad Cow Disease in a single "downer" (a non-ambulatory, disabled) dairy cow in Washington state. On December 25, this diagnosis was confirmed by a laboratory in Weybridge, England. In the wake of this shocking discovery, the Centers for Disease Control called on physicians in the United States to be aware of the clinical features of the human form of Mad Cow Disease, called variant Creutzfeldt-Jakob Disease (vCJD), and asked them to arrange for brain autopsies on all patients who died with suspected or probable vCJD to more definitely assess whether vCJD exists in the United States. Meat from the infected cow was distributed in six states, and some of it had been consumed before the USDA Food Safety and Inspection Service (FSIS) was able to recall the meat from the infected animal.[1]

Until December 23, 2003, there had never been a case of Mad Cow Disease in the United States. However, there is an epidemic of Chronic Wasting Disease in American elk and deer, involving twelve states, including a recent spread into the white-tailed deer population of Wisconsin.[2]

Abnormal prion proteins in these wild animals, when eaten by hunters, have caused the human version of Mad Cow Disease.[3]

Although it is widely believed that the deadly abnormal prion protein is confined to the brain and spinal cord, Dr. Glotzel and colleagues at the Institute of Neuropathology and National Reference Center for Prion Diseases in Zurich, Switzerland, found abnormal prion proteins in the spleen and muscle of about one-third of patients who died with sporadic CJD.[4] Thus it is possible that cattle, deer, and other wild animals infected with the deadly abnormal prion protein may harbor these infectious agents in their muscle meat.

Dr. Race at the National Institutes of Health found prions in American wild deer indistinguishable from those in mad cows.[5] And Dr. Zanusso at the University of Verona in Rome found the abnormal prion protein in the cilia hairs that hang down from the nerve that provides our sense of smell in the top of the nose.[6] Humans shed these cilia hairs every two weeks. Thus, it is possible that chronic wasting disease is spreading rapidly in deer and elk in part because prions, released into nasal secretions, are shared when these animals nuzzle each other. As deer and cattle share the same grazing land, a potential risk may exist for American cattle to be contaminated with abnormal prions from infected wild animals.

Meat from domestic animals is increasingly contaminated with bacteria, including Salmonella, toxic E.Coli, and Listeria, which can bring death to the elderly and young children,[7] and meat has been documented to transmit antibiotic resistance.[8] As animals become more diseased, so do their products. I replaced skim milk with soy milk several years ago when I learned that only fifteen seconds of 161°F heat makes the difference between pasteurized and non-pasteurized milk. Non-pasteurized milk often contains Bovine Leukemia Virus (which can cause chronic leukemia/lymphoma cancer in cows, sheep, and goats, and can cause leukemia in chimpanzees), Bovine Immunodeficiency Virus (whose major core protein is similar in shape to Human Immunodeficiency Virus), E. Coli 0157:H7 (which can cause kidney failure in children and bloody diarrhea in adults), Salmonella, and Mycobacterium Paratuberculosis (which growing evidence links to Crohn's Disease).

Eggs, too, are increasingly infected with Salmonella, putting the elderly at risk, and causing diarrhea in healthy adults and children.

Adopting a plant-based diet minimizes exposure to the above agents and just might even save your life. Remember, Creutzfeldt-Jakob disease, the human form of Mad Cow Disease, is always fatal, and there is no treatment.[9] Truly, it's time to enjoy the protection of a diet made up exclusively of plant foods.

---

[1] *Morbidity and Mortality Weekly Report,* January 9, 2004, 52(53); 1280-1285.

[2] P. Yam, "Shoot This Deer," *Scientific American,* June 2003, pp. 39-43.

[3] B. McCombie, "Deadly Venison?" *Field and Stream,* February 2001, pp. 42-45.

[4] M. Glotzel, *New England Journal of Medicine,* November 2003, 349(19): 1812-1820.

[5] R. E. Race, *Journal of Virology*, December 2002, 76 (23):12365-12368.

[6] G. Zanusso, *New England Journal of Medicine*, February, 20, 2003, 348 (8):711-719.

[7] *Morbidity and Mortality Weekly Report*, "Public Health Dispatch: Outbreak of Listeriosis—Northeastern United States," October 25, 2002, 51 (42):950-951.

[8] *Morbidity and Mortality Weekly Report*, "Outbreak of Multidrug-Resistant Salmonella Newport—United States January-April, 2002," June 28, 2002, 51 (25):545-548. T. L. Sørensen, "Transient Intestinal Carriage After Ingestion Of Antibiotic-Resistant Enterococcus Faecium From Chicken and Pork," *New England Journal of Medicine*, 2001, 345:1161-1166.

[9] S. B. Prusiner, "Shattuck Lecture—Neurodegenerative Diseases And Prions," *New England Journal of Medicine*, May 17, 2001, 344 (20):1516-1526.

CHAPTER 16

Lower Your Blood Pressure

Many today want to know how to lower their blood pressure. More than 50 percent of adult Americans, and 80 percent of those over fifty years of age, have higher than optimal blood pressure.[1] Ideal blood pressure is less than 120/80. Dr. Appleby at the University of Oxford, England, analyzed data from the study, European Prospective Investigation into Cancer and Nutrition, and discovered that vegans—those eating only plants—have the lowest blood pressure of any group studied. Only 5.8 percent of male vegans had high blood pressure, compared with 15 percent of meat eaters.[2] High blood pressure is defined as one that consistently registers 140/90 or higher.[3]

Dr. Sacks and colleagues at Harvard Medical School have found a diet that lowers blood pressure about as much as does medication. In fact, under this diet, the systolic blood pressure (the top number) dropped 11.5 points in men with high blood pressure and 7.1 points in men with normal blood pressure. Women had slightly lower reductions. To accomplish these blood pressure reductions, researchers took a meat-based diet and made it more plant-based, included nine daily servings of fruits and vegetables, and enriched the diet with calcium, using low-fat dairy products. Clearly, the more plant-based the diet, the lower the blood pressure. The lowest blood pressure is found when all animal products are removed. In fact, Dr. Rivas at the School of Medicine of Gre'teil, France has demonstrated that in one study, systolic blood pressure decreased just 1.4 points when patients drank milk, but dropped 18.4 points when patients drank soy milk.[4] Choosing foods from the Creator's original diet of fruits, whole grains, beans, vegetables, nuts, and seeds always gives the lowest blood pressure.

To optimize your blood pressure, adopt these lifestyle habits:

◆ Eat nine one-half cup servings of fruits and vegetables daily.

◆ Choose a plant-based diet.

◆ Take 500 mg to 1000 mg of calcium citrate daily.

◆ Replace meat, poultry, fish, and cheese with beans, whole grains, unsalted nuts, and seeds.

◆ Choose packaged foods with a single ingredient (i.e., rolled oats, brown rice, kidney beans, lentils, whole wheat pasta).

◆ Avoid packaged foods with "partially-hydrogenated" vegetable oil, "enriched" wheat flour, corn syrup, or salt.

◆ Walk briskly for a total of sixty minutes six days a week.

◆ Drink at least ten to twelve eight-ounce glasses of water daily.

◆ Get fifteen minutes of exposure to the sun on your face, hands, and arms at least three days a week.

◆ Consider taking 1,000 IU to 2, 000 IU of vitamin D daily.

◆ Avoid coffee, tea, colas, sodas, caffeine, and tobacco.

◆ Eat only fresh fruit or steamed above-the-ground vegetables at supper, or eat nothing at all after 3 P.M.

◆ Get seven to eight hours of sleep each night—two-and-a-half to three hours of which would be best before midnight.

These are among the Creator's chosen methods to bring about optimal blood pressure.[5]

[1] M. R. Joffres, "Distribution of Blood Pressure and Hypertension in Canada and the United States," *American Journal of Hypertension,* November 14, 2001, (11 Pt 1):1099-1105. J. Stamler, "Blood Pressure, Systolic and Diastolic, and Cardiovascular Risks. US population data," *Archives of Internal Medicine,* March 8, 1993, 153 (5):598-615.

[2] P. N. Appleby, "Hypertension and Blood Pressure Among Meat Eaters, Fish Eaters, Vegetarians and Vegans in EPIC-Oxford," *Public Health Nutrition,* 5 (5):645-654.

[3] A. V. Chobanian, "Detection, Evaluation, and Treatment of High Blood Pressure: The JNC 7 Report," *Journal of the American Medical Association,* 2003, 289:2560-2572.

[4] M. Rivas, "Soy Milk Lowers Blood Pressure in Men and Women With Mild to Moderate Essential Hypertension," *Journal of Nutrition,* 132:1900-1902.

[5] See E. G. White, *The Ministry of Healing,* p. 127, and *Counsels on Diet and Foods,* p. 301.

CHAPTER 17

Reduce Your Risk of Cancer

Cancer is the number two killer of Americans. However, the American Cancer Society estimates that one-third of cancer cases is related to poor diet and another third to cigarette smoking. Therefore, two-thirds of cancer cases are potentially preventable. In addition, for those who do not smoke, diet and exercise are the most powerful tools available to prevent cancer.

Recently, the American Institute for Cancer Research and the World Cancer Research Fund launched a second comprehensive review of the scientific literature regarding the role of diet and nutrition in lowering the risk of cancer. Twenty researchers from twelve countries will review 10,000 scientific studies and report their findings in 2006. The information in the rest of this chapter is based on the report of the last such review, released in 1997.[1] According to this report, 30 percent to 40 percent of cancer cases worldwide—some three to four million cases annually—are preventable with proper diet, exercise, and optimal weight. Specifically, 20 percent to 33 percent of lung cancer cases in both smokers and nonsmokers may be prevented with a diet high in fruits and vegetables.

The researchers also found that 66 percent to 75 percent of stomach cancer may be prevented with a diet high in vegetables and fruits and low in salt and salted foods. The research panel also found that a plant-based diet, along with avoiding alcohol, maintaining healthy weight, and regular exercise, may decrease the risk of breast cancer by 33 percent to 50 percent. However, these habits must be in place from puberty into adult life to obtain maximal protection.

The report notes as well that diets high in vegetables and low in meat, in conjunction with regular exercise and abstaining from alcohol may lower the risk of colon cancer by 66 percent to 75 percent. Backing up these findings are the results of the European Prospective Investigation into Cancer (EPIC) study tracking over half a million Europeans in twelve countries for four and a half years showing that those eating the highest amounts of fiber were at a 40 percent lower risk of colon cancer than those eating the least amount.[2] Since only plants contain dietary fiber, those eating the most plant food have the lowest risk of colon cancer.

The American Institute for Cancer Research report also found that a diet high in vegetables and fruits, while avoiding alcohol, may prevent 33 percent to 50 percent of cancers of the mouth and pharynx. Finally, this expert panel determined that avoiding food contaminated with aflatoxins and abstaining from alcohol may prevent 33 percent to 66 percent of liver cancers.

Scientists with the AICR give the following recommendations for lowering your risk of cancer:

- Choose a plant-based diet rich in vegetables, fruit, beans, and whole grains.
- Eat five servings of vegetables and fruits daily.
- Eat seven or more servings daily of whole grains, beans, root vegetables.
- Avoid refined sugar.
- Avoid meat, especially red meat.
- Restrict dietary fat to no more than 15 percent of total calories consumed.
- Avoid processed oils.
- Take in no more than one teaspoon of salt daily.
- Refrigerate leftover food immediately.
- Avoid food containing additives and residues.
- Do not eat charred, broiled, cured, or smoked meats.
- Exercise vigorously at least one hour a week.
- Take a brisk walk for one hour daily.
- Keep Body Mass Index (BMI) at 21 to 23.
- Gain no more than eleven pounds in adulthood.
- Do not consume alcohol.
- Do not smoke or chew tobacco.

---

[1] J. Potter, Chair, Expert Panel of the Diet and Cancer Project, Executive summary of "Food, Nutrition and the Prevention of Cancer: A Global Perspective," American Institute for Cancer Research/World Cancer Research Fund, 1997.

[2] S. A. Bingham, "Dietary Fibre in Food and Protection Against Colorectal Cancer in the European Prospective Investigation into Cancer and Nutrition (EPIC): An Observational Study," *The Lancet*, 2003, 361:1496-501.

CHAPTER 18

Medicine for the Mind

Let's consider tools to help fight depression. Increasing serotonin in the brain helps improve mood and relieves depression. Serotonin is made from the amino acid tryptophan. Adequate dietary tryptophan helps improve mood. Dr. Smith at Littlemore Hospital, Oxford, England found that 67 percent of patients with depression relapsed into significant depressive symptoms when tryptophan was removed from their diet.[1]

Dr. Wurtman of the Massachusetts Institute of Technology found that a diet rich in carbohydrates, increased available tryptophan by as much as 54 percent by limiting the intake of five competing amino acids.[2] Because only plants contain carbohydrates, a plant diet increases tryptophan and thus helps raise serotonin.

Vitamin B_6 is also needed to make serotonin. Dr. Bernstein reported in the *Annals of the New York Academy of Science* that vitamin B_6 has been observed to raise serotonin levels.[3] Dr. Alpert, Harvard Medical School, has found that 15 percent to 38 percent of adults with depression have low blood folic acid levels.[4] And Dr. Teimeier of the Erasmus Medical Center in Rotterdam, Netherlands, found patients with depression had low levels of vitamin B_{12} and folic acid.[5]

Another factor in increasing serotonin levels is bright light. Dr. Lambert at the Baker Heart Research Institute in Melbourne, Australia, found that brain serotonin levels were eight times higher on a bright day than on an overcast day.[6] Dr. Oren at Yale University found depression scores cut in half when women suffering from depression following the birth of a child (postpartum depression) were treated with three weeks of bright light.[7] And Dr. Leppamaki of the National Public Health Institute in Finland found bright light reduced depression symptoms even more than exercise.[8] Dr. Terman at Columbia University found bright light *and* negative ions (found in fresh air) together improved depression symptoms in those with Seasonal Affective Disorder.[9]

Dr. Kennedy at the University of New Orleans found exercise—espcially high-intensity exercise—reduced tension, depression, fatigue, and anger.[10]

So, to help improve your mood and combat depression:

- ◆ Eat a plant-based diet, which helps raise serotonin levels.
- ◆ Maximize tryptophan levels by eating soy beans, pumpkin seeds, sesame seeds, almonds, and beans.
- ◆ Get thirty minutes of exposure to bright sunlight in the morning or take two fifteen-minute walks outdoors between 9:00 A.M. and 3:00 P.M. daily. Be careful never to burn your skin. Only your eyes need exposure to sunlight in order to raise serotonin, so you can keep your skin covered, as necessary, to prevent sunburn.

- Walk briskly for one hour six days a week.
- Eat one to two tablespoons of freshly ground flaxseed daily (measure tablespoons of the whole seeds and then grind in a coffee grinder).
- Eat one ounce (a cupped handful) of English walnuts at breakfast and lunch until symptoms of depression subside, then one ounce of nuts daily.
- Take a B-complex vitamin at the noon or evening meal.
- Dismiss negative thoughts and speak nothing negative of others.

[1] K. A. Smith, *The Lancet*, March 29, 1997, 349 (9056):915-919.

[2] R. J. Wurtman, *American Journal of Clinical Nutrition*, 2003, 77:128-132.

[3] A. L. Bernstein, *Annals of The New York Academy of Science*, 190, 585:250-260.

[4] J. E. Alpert, *Nutritional Review*, May 1997, 55 (5):145-149.

[5] H. Tiemeier, *American Journal of Psychiatry*, December 2002, 159 (12):2099-2101.

[6] G. W. Lambert, *The Lancet*, December 2002, 360 (9348):1840-1842.

[7] D. A. Oren, *American Journal of Psychiatry*, April 2002, 159 (4):666-669.

[8] S. J. Leppamaki, *Journal of Clinical Psychiatry*, April 2002, 63 (4):316-321.

[9] M. Terman, *Archives of General Psychiatry*, October 1998, 55 (10):875-882.

[10] M. M. Kennedy, *Journal of Sports Medicine and Physical Fitness*, September, 37 (3):200-204.

CHAPTER 19

Live Heart Healthy

In America, heart disease cuts short more lives every year—nearly 750,000—than any other medical problem. The major underlying cause of heart disease is atherosclerosis, the buildup of cholesterol in the walls of the coronary arteries. And cigarette smoking and insulin resistance accelerate atherosclerosis.[1] Obviously, one excellent way to reduce your risk of heart disease is to stop smoking—or avoid taking up the habit. You can help combat insulin resistance by choosing foods with a low glycemic index. Such foods include apples, pears, apricots, plums, peaches, cherries, blueberries, beans, leafy greens, above-the-ground vegetables, oats, barley, rye, nuts, and seeds.

In spite of the high rate of heart disease in America today, Dr. Stampfer and colleagues at the Harvard School of Public Health have found a group of Americans at 82 percent lower risk of heart attack than all other Americans.[2] Their secrets? They do not smoke, keep their body mass index (BMI) under 25 (based on optimal weight for one's height), walk briskly at least thirty minutes daily, and eat generously of whole grains, omega-3 fats (best eaten in flaxseed, English walnuts, and dark leafy greens), and folic acid (found in beans and dark leafy greens). They also eat more plant food than most Americans, eat the least "partially hydrogenated" vegetable oil (found in baked goods, margarine, and fried foods), and they eat diets high in those foods least likely to raise blood sugar—such as beans, above-the-ground vegetables, northern fruits (ie. apples, pears, peaches, cherries, plums, apricots, berries), steamed whole grains, unsalted nuts, and seeds.

Dr. William Castelli, Medical Director of the Framingham Cardiovascular Institute, directed the longest ongoing heart study in the United States. He directed the Framingham heart study for twenty years, and during its course, he never saw anyone in the study have a heart attack if that person's total cholesterol level remained below 150.[3] In contrast, he found that 35 percent of all heart attacks in this country occur in Americans whose total cholesterol runs between 150 and 200. Dr. Roberts at the Pritikin Longevity Center recently demonstrated that Americans can bring their total cholesterol from an average of 191 to 154 in just three weeks using a diet consisting of nearly 100 percent plant foods.[4] Specifically, this diet was made up of 10 percent calories from fat, 15 percent to 20 percent calories from protein, 70 percent to 75 percent calories primarily from unrefined carbohydrates, five or more servings per day of whole grains, four or more servings per day of vegetables, three or more servings per day of fruits, protein that came almost entirely from plant sources, and no alcohol, tobacco, or caffeine.[5]

If you have been struggling as a vegetarian to lower your total cholesterol levels, consider moving away from milk, eggs, and cheese. Dr. Toohey and colleagues reported their findings that the average total cholesterol of vegetarians using dairy products was 174, however, among vegetarians who left off dairy products, total cholesterol averaged 145, or less than 150.[6]

Dr. Caldwell Esselstyn, surgeon at the Cleveland Clinic, formulated a program to eliminate coronary disease and found eighteen patients with blockages in all three coronary arteries who were willing to participate in the study. Most had already failed coronary by-pass surgery or angioplasty. Together, these patients had had forty-nine coronary events in the previous eight years; their average total cholesterol was 237. Dr. Esselstyn put each patient on a diet of whole grains, beans, legumes, vegetables, and fruits. He also allowed unsalted nuts and seeds as condiments, but no oils, dairy foods, meat, poultry, or fish. After five years, none experienced any worsening of their coronary disease. Eleven patients elected to repeat a coronary angiogram, and 73 percent of the eighteen experienced some reversal of coronary blockages. No patient had a heart attack or other coronary event during twelve years, despite the group's having had forty-nine coronary events in the previous eight years. Their average total cholesterol was 145, however, Dr. Esselstyn used medication, as needed, so that all eighteen patients brought their total cholesterol below 150.[7]

When it comes to fighting coronary heart disease, a heart-healthy diet and a total cholesterol level below 150 may be all you will need.

---

[1] H. C. McGill, "Obesity Accelerates the Progression of Coronary Atherosclerosis in Young Men," *Circulation*, 2002, 105:2712-2718. E. Cho, "A Prospective Study of Obesity and Risk of Coronary Heart Disease Among

Diabetic Women," *Diabetes Care*, July 2002, 25 (7):1142-1148. D. Waters, "Effects of Cigarette Smoking on the Angiographic Evolution of Coronary Atherosclerosis: A Canadian Coronary Atherosclerosis Intervention Trial (CCAIT) Substudy" *Circulation*, 1996, 94:614-621. W. K. Al-Delaimy, "Smoking and Risk of Coronary Heart Disease Among Women With Type 2 Diabetes Mellitus," *Archives of Internal Medicine*, February 11, 2002, 162 (3):273-279.

[2] M. J. Stampfer,"Primary Prevention Of Coronary Heart Disease In Women Through Diet And Lifestyle," *New England Journal of Medicine*, 2000, 343:16-22.

[3] W. Castelli, Framingham Heart Study, quoted in *Newsweek*, November 19, 1984.

[4] C. K. Roberts, "Effect of Diet and Exercise Intervention on Blood Pressure, Insulin, Oxidative Stress, and Nitric Oxide Availability," *Circulation*, 2002, 106:2530.

[5] Ibid.

[6] M. L. Toohey, "Cardiovascular Disease Risk Factors are Lower in African-American Vegans Compared to Lacto-Ovo-Vegetarians," *Journal of the American College of Nutrition*, October 1998, 17 (5):425-434.

[7] C. B. Esselstyn, "Resolving the Coronary Artery Disease Epidemic Through Plant-Based Nutrition," *Prev Cardiology*, Autumn 2001, 4 (4):171-177. "Updating a 12-Year Experience With Arrest and Reversal Therapy for Coronary Heart Disease (An Overdue Requiem for Palliative Cardiology)," *American Journal of Cardiology*, August 1, 1999, 84 (3):339-341, A8. "Changing the Treatment Paradigm for Coronary Artery Disease," *American Journal of Cardiology*, November 26, 1998, 82 (10B):2T-4T. "A Strategy to Arrest and Reverse Coronary Artery Disease: A 5-Year Longitudinal Study of a Single Physician's Practice," *Journal of Family Practice*, December 1995, 41 (6):560-568.

CHAPTER 20

Keep Insulin Levels Low

If you want optimal health, keep your insulin level low. Excess weight raises insulin. Insulin can stimulate cell growth and may promote cancer. In fact, one report indicates that the heaviest Americans are at a 52 percent to 62 percent higher risk of dying from cancer than those of normal weight.[1] To lose weight, eat for breakfast only 100 percent whole grain cereal (especially hot cereal), northern fruits, and a handful of unsalted nuts. For lunch, eat soupy, savory beans poured over steamed 100 percent whole grains, steamed and raw vegetables, topped with tomato puree, humus, or cashew sauce, and small amounts of olives or avocado. Eat nothing after 3 P.M.—or just an apple or moderate quantities of fresh fruit or a plate of steamed vegetables for supper. Gradually work up to a brisk walk for a total of one hour daily, as you are able and only if your doctor approves.

Furthermore, to keep insulin low, avoid highly processed food and foods that more easily raise blood sugar. Dr. Michaud and colleagues at the National Cancer Institute found that overweight individuals who ate foods containing the least amount of fructose and foods not as prone to raise blood sugar had one-half to one-third the pancreatic cancer risk of those eating foods with greater ability to raise blood sugar.[2]

Similarly, Dr. Franceschi and colleagues reported in the *Annals of Oncology* that people eating foods that raised blood sugar the most had a 70 percent to 80 percent higher risk of colon cancer as those avoiding such foods.[3] And a study at the Harvard Medical School found that individuals eating foods high in the ability to raise blood sugar were at nearly three times greater risk of coronary artery disease compared to those avoiding these foods.[4]

Another study indicated that when patients with diabetes chose foods with the least ability to raise blood sugar, they experienced as much as a 27 percent drop in the amount of sugar bound to blood protein.[5] The same report listed those foods most potent at raising blood sugar. Individuals eating generously of these foods were found to be most likely to develop type 2 diabetes. These foods included French fries, potato chips, white bread, white rice, pasta, white potatoes, cola beverages, and sweetened beverages—both carbonated and noncarbonated. Therefore, to lower the risk of cancer, heart attack, and diabetes, avoid these foods. Also, if a packaged food has more than one ingredient, leave it in the store. This is the message I give my patients at Lifestyle Center of America.

[1] E. E. Calle, "Overweight, Obesity, and Mortality From Cancer in a Prospectively studied Cohort of U.S. Adults," *New England Journal of Medicine*, April 2003, 348 (17):1625-1638.

[2] "Dietary Sugar, Glycemic Load, and Pancreatic Cancer Risk in a Prospective Study," *Journal of the National Cancer Institute*, September 4, 2002, 94 (17):1293-1300.

[3] S. Franceschi, "Dietary Glycemic Load and Colorectal Cancer Risk," *Annals of Oncology,* February 2001, 12 (2):173-178.

[4] S. Liu, "A Prospective Study of Dietary Glycemic Load, Carbohydrate Intake, and Risk of Coronary Heart Disease in US Women," *American Journal of Clinical Nutrition,* June 2000, 71 (6):1455-1461.

[5] W. Willett, "Glycemic Index, Glycemic Load, and Risk of Type 2 Diabetes," *American Journal of Clinical Nutrition,* 2002, 76 (Suppl):274S-280S.

CHAPTER 21

Protect Your Prostate

In looking at prostate cancer, let's consider some encouraging data.

Dr. Brooks and colleagues at Duke University found that men with high selenium levels were at a 76 percent lower risk of prostate cancer than were men with the lowest selenium levels.[1]

Dr. Jacobsen of Loma Linda University found that men drinking soy milk more than once a day were at a 70 percent lower risk of prostate cancer than men who rarely or never drank soy milk.[2]

Dr. Ahonen reported in the journal *Cancer Causes and Control* that men with high levels of vitamin D were at less than one-third the risk of prostate cancer of men with the lowest levels of vitamin D in their blood.[3]

Another study reported that those men with the smallest waistlines and lowest insulin levels had a risk of prostate cancer only 12 percent that of those men with the largest waistlines and the highest insulin levels.[4]

Dr. Giovannucci reported in the *Journal of the National Cancer Institute* that men eating more than ten servings of tomato a week were at a 35 percent lower risk of prostate cancer than were men who ate less than one and a half servings a week.[5]

Dr. Chan reported a study in which those men using the fewest dairy products were at a 34 percent lower risk of prostate cancer than were those men eating the most dairy products.[6]

And finally, Dr. Reichman conducted a study in which those men with the highest vitamin A levels had less than half the prostate cancer risk of the men with the lowest vitamin A levels.[7]

Based on these studies, the following guidelines can help you lower your risk of prostate cancer:

- Use tomato puree generously. (Tomato puree is one of the few tomato products with no added salt.)
- Eat three Brazil nuts daily (400 mcg of selenium).
- Choose only 100 percent whole grains.
- Use soy milk instead of cow's milk.
- Use cashew or tofu-based sauces in place of cheese.
- Spend about fifteen minutes in direct sunlight daily even on cloudy days. Be very careful never to burn your skin with excessive sunlight exposure!
- Take 1,000 IU to 2,000 IU of vitamin D total daily, no more.
- Eat generously of cruciferous vegetables.
- Choose orange and yellow fruits and vegetables.
- Have an annual prostate exam and PSA after age fifty.

---

[1] J. D. Brooks, "Plasma Selenium Level Before Diagnosis and the Risk of Prostate Cancer Development," *The Journal of Urology,* 2001 166:2034-2038.

[2] B. K. Jacobsen, "Does High Soy Milk Intake Reduce Prostate Cancer

Incidence? The Adventist Health Study (United States)," *Cancer Causes and Control,* 9 (6):553-557.

[3] M. H. Ahonen, "Prostate Cancer Risk and Prediagnostic Serum 25-Hydroxyvitamin D Levels (Finland)," *Cancer Causes and Control,* October 11, 2000, (9):847-852.

[4] A. W. Hsing, "Insulin Resistance and Prostate Cancer Risk," *Journal of the National Cancer Institute,* January 2003, 95 (1):67-71.

[5] E. Giovannucci, "Intake of Carotenoids and Retinol in Relation to Risk of Prostate Cancer," *Journal of the National Cancer Institute,* December 6, 1995, 87 (23):1767-1776.

[6] J. M. Chan, "Dairy Products, Calcium, and Prostate Cancer Risk in the Physicians' Health Study," *American Journal of Clinical Nutrition,* October 2001, 74 (4):549-554.

[7] M. E. Reichman, "Serum Vitamin A and Subsequent Development of Prostate Cancer in the First National Health and Nutrition Examination Survey Epidemiologic Follow-up Study," *Cancer Research,* April 15, 1990, 50 (8):2311-2315.

CHAPTER 22

Abstain From Alcohol

Alcohol is toxic to the nerves and interferes with protein receptors on the nerve membranes, actually impairing nerve impulses and frontal lobe functions such as judgment and willpower. In effect, alcohol can give one a chemical frontal lobotomy, thus, leaving one under the control of the passions, drives, and desires, rather than under the control of reason.[1] This is part of the reason that each year nearly one in four victims of violent crime report that the offender had been drinking alcohol prior committing the crime.[2] Among attacks committed by a current or former intimate partner of the victim, two out of three offenders had been drinking prior to the attack.[3]

Dr. Foster at Columbia University found that half of the nation's alcohol is consumed either by underage drinkers or by adults consuming excessive amounts of alcohol.[4] Further, Dr. Naimi at the Centers for Disease Control and Prevention found that nearly half of all binge drinking episodes occur among non-heavy drinkers. In fact, 73 percent of binge drinkers were moderate drinkers, and 69 percent of binge-drinking episodes occurred among those twenty-six years of age and older—not among the youngest drinkers. Binge drinkers were fourteen times more likely to drive impaired by alcohol than were nonbinge drinkers.[5] Dr. Zador found that male drivers sixteen to twenty years old driving with a blood alcohol level between 0.08 percent and 0.1 percent (within the legal limit in several states) were at fifty-two times greater risk of death in a single vehicle car accident than was a youth without alcohol in his blood.[6]

Women are especially vulnerable to the toxic effects of alcohol. Dr. Beral of Oxford, England, reports that women consuming three alcohol drinks daily were at a 46 percent greater risk of breast cancer than non-drinkers and that breast cancer risk increased 7.1 percent with each additional alcoholic beverage consumed.[7]

Perhaps those most vulnerable to the damaging effects of alcohol are the unborn. Dr. Kesmodel at Aarhus University Hospital in Denmark found that pregnant women consuming five or more alcohol drinks per week were at nearly three times the risk of experiencing a still birth.[8]

According to the "Tenth Special Report on Alcohol and Health to the U.S. Congress," alcohol is second only to Alzheimer's disease as a cause of adult dementia. Prolonged exposure to alcohol results in loss of brain nerve cells. In severe cases, this loss of brain mass can be seen with an MRI.[9] However, one drink is all that is needed to bring *chemical* changes that may never be seen with sophisticated brain imaging devices.[10]

I remember a patient in a substance abuse treatment program during my residency. He never had planned to use hard street drugs, like cocaine, but after drinking alcohol, when offered harder drugs, he had no will-power to say "No," and thus ended up abusing drugs.

Alcohol is detrimental to health and can be highly addictive. But remember, your Creator wants to help you conquer your addictions. Focus your attention on Him by spending quality time with Him. Give yourself over to His daily care. And He will guide you to freedom.

[1] B. J. Flanigan, "Alcohol Use, Sexual Intercourse, and an Exploratory Study," *Journal of Alcohol Drug Education,* Spring 1986, 31 (3):6-40. K. Fromme, "Intoxicated Sexual Risk Taking: An Expectancy or Cognitive Impairment Explanation?," *Journal of the Study of Alcohol,* January 1999, 60 (1):54-63. R. J. MacGowan, "Predictors of Risky Sex of Young Men After Release From Prison," *International Journal of Sexually Transmitted Diseases and AIDS,* August 2003, 14 (8):519-523. D. Giacopassi, "An Analysis of the Relationship of Alcohol to Casino Gambling Among College Students," *Journal of Gambling Studies,* Summer 1998, 14 (2):135-149.

[2] D. E. Shalala, E, Gordis, "Tenth Special Report to the U.S. Congress on Alcohol and Health," U.S. Department of Health and Human Services, Public Health Service, National Institutes of Health, National Institute on Alcohol Abuse and Alcoholism, June 2000, chapter 2, p. 54.

[3] Ibid.

[4] S. E. Foster, "Alcohol Consumption and Expenditures for Underage Drinking and Adult Excessive Drinking," *Journal of the American Medical Association,* February 26, 2003, 289 (8):989-995.

[5] T. S. Naimi, "Binge Drinking Among US Adults," *Journal of the American Medical Association,* January 1, 2003, 289 (1):70-75.

[6] P. L. Zador, "Alcohol-Related Relative Risk of Driver Fatalities and Driver Involvement in Fatal Crashes in Relation to Driver Age and Gender: An Update Using 1996 Data," *Journal of the Study of Alcohol,* May 2000, 61 (3):387-395.

[7] V. Beral, "Alcohol, Tobacco and Breast cancer—Collaborative Reanalysis of Individual Data From 53 Epidemiological Studies, Including 58,515 Women With Breast Cancer and 95,067 Women Without the Disease," *British Journal of Cancer,* November, 18, 2002, 87 (11):1234-1245.

[8] U. Kesmodel, "Moderate Alcohol Intake During Pregnancy and the Risk of Stillbirth and Death in the First Year of Life," *American Journal of Epidemiology,* February 15, 2002, 155 (4):305-312.

[9] D. E. Shalala, E. Gordis, "Tenth Special Report to the U.S. Congress on Alcohol and Health," U.S. Department of Health and Human Services, Public Health Service, National Institutes of Health, National Institute on Alcohol Abuse and Alcoholism, June 2000, chapter 2, pp. 134, 135.

[10] N. Nedley, *Proof Positive: How to Reliably Combat Disease and Achieve Optimal Health Through Nutrition and Lifestyle* (Ardmore, OK: Nedley Publishing, 1999), CD-ROM Version, Record 4,725/6,450, Hit 3/6.

CHAPTER 23

It Pays to Quit Smoking

Let's look at some great reasons to quit smoking.

Dr. Dobson at Royal Newcastle Hospital in Australia found that women who smoked were five times more likely to have a heart attack than non-smoking women. But he also found that three years after they quit smoking, their risk of having a heart attack had decreased so that it was equal to that of non-smokers![1] Likewise, at the University of Newcastle, Dr. McElduff found a dramatic drop in the risk of heart attack for both men and women after just one to three years without cigarettes.[2]

Dr. Rea at the University of Seattle found that for smokers who survived a heart attack and then quit smoking the risk of a second heart attack decreased from being 50 percent greater than non-smokers to the same risk as non-smokers after just three years.[3] Other reports indicate that twenty years after quitting, a former smoker's risk of lung cancer is just one-fourth that of a current smoker.[4]

Dr. Fuchs at Brigham and Women's Hospital, Boston found that the risk of pancreatic cancer was cut in half just two years after quitting smoking.[5] Dr. Wannamethee at the Royal Free Hospital School of Medicine in London found stroke risk dropped by more than half in smokers who quit.[6] Hospital admissions for chronic bronchitis and emphysema dropped by 43 percent for smokers who quit smoking, according to one study in Denmark.[7] In a French study, researchers discovered that the risk of bladder cancer in ex-smokers dropped by 80 percent twenty-five years after they quite smoking.[8]

Finally, Dr. Chao at the American Cancer Society found that the longer you are without cigarettes, the lower your risk of colon cancer.[9]

Truly, it pays to quit smoking. If you have tried to quit smoking and found it difficult, here are a few tips to help:

- Set a firm date to quit.
- Quit all at once; don't try to taper off.
- Eat only fresh fruit and 100 percent fruit juice for the first two or three days after quitting.
- Eat a plant-based diet thereafter.
- Drink ten to twelve eight-ounce glasses of water daily between meals.
- Leave off caffeine and alcohol for life!
- Eat very light evening meals.
- Take a daily B-complex vitamin for one or two weeks after quitting.
- Switch to 100 percent whole-grain breads and cereals.
- Take a walk after meals—especially a large meal.
- When a strong craving for tobacco comes, take deep, slow breaths, using the diaphragm muscle, drink a glass of water, or take a brief walk.
- Avoid places and situations where you used to smoke.

- Spend a thoughtful hour with your Creator the first thing every morning to become better acquainted with Him as a real Person and a real Friend.
- Turn over your habit to Him each day; ask for His divine power to help you overcome your addictive habit(s).
- Avoid doing anything that would make it easier for you to return to smoking.

[1] A. J. Dobson, "How Soon After Quitting Smoking Does Risk of Heart Attack Decline?" *Journal of Clinical Epidemiolody*, 1991, 44 (11):1247-1253.

[2] P. McElduff, "Rapid Reduction in Coronary Risk for Those Who Quit Cigarette Smoking," *Australian/New Zealand Journal of Public Health*, December 1998, 22 (7):787-791.

[3] T. D. Rea, "Smoking Status and Risk for Recurrent Coronary Events After Myocardial Infarction," *Annals of Internal Medicine*, September 2002, 137 (6):494-500.

[4] H. Pohlabeln, "The Relation Between Various Histological Types of Lung Cancer and the Number of Years Since Cessation of Smoking," *Lung Cancer*, November 1997, 18 (3):223-229.

[5] C. S. Fuchs, "A Prospective Study of Cigarette Smoking and the Risk of Pancreatic Cancer," *Archives of Internal Medicine*, October 1996, 156 (19):2255-2260.

[6] S. G. Wannamethee, "Smoking Cessation and the Risk of Stroke in Middle-Aged Men," *Journal of the American Medical Association*, July 1995, 274 (2):155-160.

[7] N. S. Godtfredsen, "Risk of Hospital Admission for COPD Following Smoking Cessation and Reduction: A Danish Population Study," *Thorax*, November 2002, 57 (11):967-972.

[8] P. Brennan, "Cigarette Smoking and Bladder Cancer in Men: A Pooled Analysis of 11 Case-Control Studies," *International Journal of Cancer*, April 2000, 86 (2):289-294.

[9] A. Chao, "Cigarette Smoking and Colorectal Cancer Mortality in the Cancer Prevention Study II," *Journal of the National Cancer Institute*, December 2000, 92 (23):1888-1896.

CHAPTER 24

Lifestyle Changes That Last

Have you struggled unsuccessfully to stop harmful habits or found it difficult to adopt healthier ones? There is hope. Daily take full advantage of this law of the Universe: By beholding we become changed (see 2 Corinthians 3:18).

I was eating breakfast with my oldest daughter Jena when she was about two years of age. I was in a hurry, so when nothing remained in my cereal bowl but soymilk, I decided to use my bowl as a glass and quickly drank the milk right from the bowl! Moments later, to my surprise and great dismay, I saw my daughter raise her bowl and drink from it just like Daddy. I had never seen her do that before. I was about to scold her when I suddenly realized that by beholding she had become changed.

The question, then, is: What do we behold? The owner's manual has the answer: "Behold the Lamb of God, which taketh away the sin of the world" (John 1:29). These were the words spoken about the Savior when He stepped onto the world stage, and they contain the secret to lasting lifestyle change. As we behold our Creator, the Lamb of God, we are changed to be like Him. What happened to the Lamb? It was killed (see Exodus 12:21-27). If you want to be forever separated from destructive lifestyle habits, study the Savior's life and death. If you have been struggling without success to make lasting changes in your life, try spending a thoughtful hour every morning studying the closing scenes of the Savior's life. "Let the imagination vividly grasp each scene."[1] Study the character of your Creator. Spend time alone at the beginning of every day contemplating the life of the Son of man through His Word and through prayer. Become better acquainted with Him as a real Person and a real Friend. Every morning officially invite Him to tackle your most destructive lifestyle habits, to live inside you and rule you.

As you behold your Creator, you will become like Him. You will also be strengthened to bear trials and to make changes in your lifestyle that last. If you're struggling to make permanent lifestyle changes, let me make a suggestion. Keep close to the Savior. Spend time in communication with your Creator. You will find He keeps your lifestyle on track as you stay connected with Him.

---

[1] E. G. White, *Gospel Workers* (Hagerstown, Md.: Review and Herald), p. 246.

Changing Lifestyles ... Restoring Health

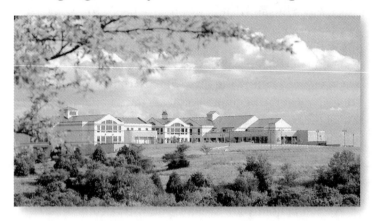

For free information about the Lifestyle Center of America and our life changing 11-day and 17-day Health Restoration Programs for:

- Diabetes
- Heart Disease
- Hypertension
- Excess Weight
- Other chronic degenerative diseases

Call 800-213-8955 or visit our website at
www.lifestylecenter.org

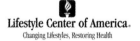

Lifestyle Center of America
Changing Lifestyles, Restoring Health

Goddard Youth Camp Road, Box 4001
Sulphur, OK 73086